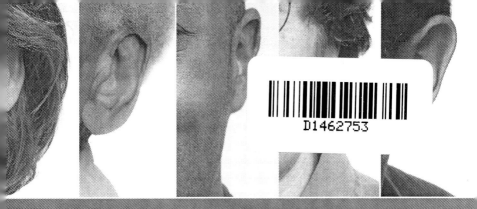

D1462753

The Hearing Aid Decision
Answers To Your Many Questions

by Randall D. Smith, M.Ed.
Jerome G. Alpiner, Ph.D.
Megan Mulvey, BA

First Edition

Published by:
Ramie Publishing Corporation
3110 S. Wadsworth Blvd., Ste. 107
Denver, Colorado 80227-4809

Copyright ©2007 by Randall D. Smith

Library of Congress Cataloging in Publication Data
Smith, Randall D.
The Hearing Aid Decision Answers to Your Many Questions/by Randall D. Smith, Jerome G. Alpiner, and
Megan Mulvey - First Edition

Library of Congress Catalog No. 2001012345

ISBN-13 978-0-9628891-0-3
ISBN-10 0-9628891-0-5

Almost everything we do in
our day-to-day life involves
communication.

Special thanks
to Sharon Alpiner Cutler and Jessea Wilson
for their keen editing skills and to
Wendy Driscoll for her layout design
in the creation of this booklet.

Preface

This book is designed for people who do not hear well. These people could be teachers, homemakers, bankers, lawyers, miners, doctors. They could be anybody, because hearing loss is not a respecter of age, gender, or economic status.

Stop and think for moment. Do you know anyone who does not hear well? It could be someone who always asks others to repeat what was said. Do YOU ask people to repeat? Have you thought that people were mumbling or not speaking loud enough? Do you say to yourself, "I hear you, but I don't understand all of the words?" Do people ever accuse you of hearing only what you want to hear--when you want to hear it? If this is the case and you do have a hearing problem, you are not alone. We don't know exactly how many hearing impaired people there are in the United States, but estimates indicate that about 30 million have a significant degree of hearing loss. We also know that hearing loss increases with age. In fact, the two most common causes of hearing loss are aging and noise exposure.

Almost everything we do in our day-to-day life involves communication. It has been said that, "Human communication is action; it is culture, it is the history of man, it is the fabric of all societies, its absence negates man's existence." (Toubbeh, J. I., Human Communication Disorders. Rehabilitation Record. 1-4 May-June, 1973).

Only a few years ago, popular belief was that hearing aids could not help people with sensorineural hearing loss (previously referred to as "nerve type") resulting, for example, from the aging process or noise exposure. The fact is, hearing aids often help those with sensorineural hearing loss. There are also many individuals who have a conductive

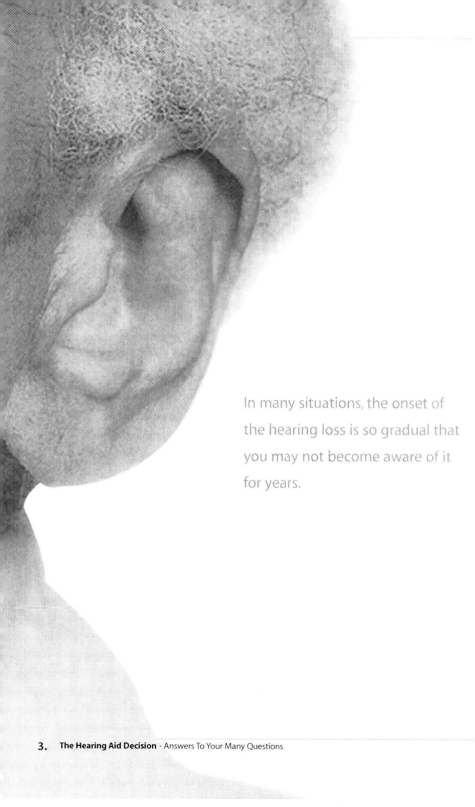

In many situations, the onset of the hearing loss is so gradual that you may not become aware of it for years.

hearing loss which may be medically treatable, for example, due to an ear infection. Sometimes, medical treatment may not be able to reverse the conductive problem, but hearing aids may help.

Are you one of those people who need hearing aids but are not using them?

Hearing loss is a hidden handicap. There are no visible clues to indicate its presence. In many situations, the onset of the hearing loss is so gradual that you may not become aware of it for years. Once the hearing loss is recognized, where do you turn for help?

Once you realize you don't hear as well as you should, there can be confusion and lack of understanding about where you can get help. This book will help you start down the path to better hearing and improved communication in your everyday life.

It is up to you to follow through for better hearing.

Jerome G. Alpiner, Ph.D.,*
Fellow, American Speech-Language -Hearing Association

---

* Alpiner, Jerome G. and Patricia A. McCarthy, Rehabilitative Audiology: Children and Adults, Third Edition, 2000, Williams and Wilkins, Baltimore.

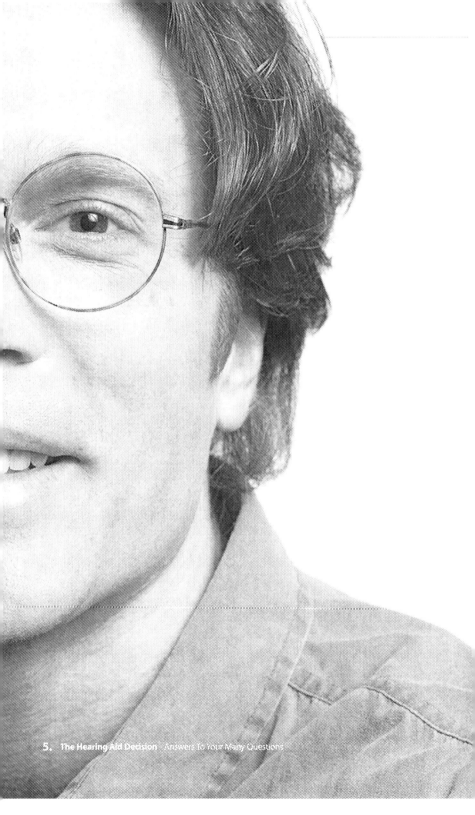

Table of Contents

Chapter 1   Let's Get Started   p. 8

Chapter 2   How's My Hearing?   p. 10

Chapter 3   Caring For Your Ears   p. 18

Chapter 4   Hearing Aid Basics   p. 20

Chapter 5   The Hearing Aid Decision   p. 26

Chapter 6   Now What?   p. 32

Chapter 7   Purchasing Your Hearing Aids   p. 38

Chapter 8   Hearing Aid Care and Maintenance   p. 42

Chapter 9   Adjusting to Your New Hearing Aids   p. 44

Chapter 10   About That Ringing and Buzzing in My Ears (Tinnitus)   p. 50

Chapter 11   Conclusion   p. 54

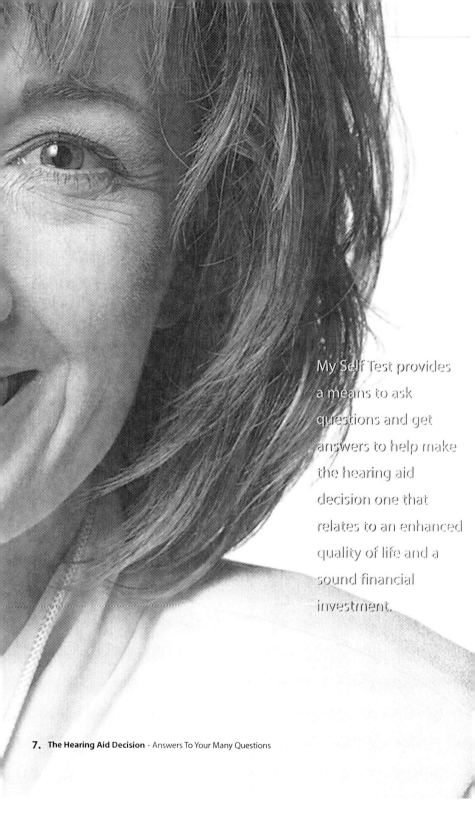

My Self Test provides a means to ask questions and get answers to help make the hearing aid decision one that relates to an enhanced quality of life and a sound financial investment.

Chapter 1

Let's Get Started

*W*elcome to The Hearing Aid Decision. Within the following pages are clear and concise answers to the many questions you may have when considering if you or a significant other would benefit from hearing amplification and how to make a smart hearing aid purchasing decision.*

Prior to writing this book, we thought it would be appropriate to survey hearing aid users (new and continuing) and individuals considering amplification to find out what was on their minds. We wanted to understand their concerns before and after their hearing aid(s) purchase. My Self Test, below, provides a means to ask questions and get answers to help make the HEARING AID DECISION one that relates to an enhanced quality of life and a sound financial investment. As you begin, take a moment to complete the following self evaluation.

My Self Test

Do I often miss what I want to hear?	YES___ NO___
Do I frequently ask people to repeat themselves?	YES___ NO___
Do I think most people mumble?	YES___ NO___
Do I strain to hear what others are saying?	YES___ NO___
Do I often misunderstand what people say?	YES___ NO___
Do I hear speech sounds, but not understand all of the words?	YES___ NO___
Do I avoid social activities because of my hearing?	YES___ NO___
Do I have trouble understanding people in noisy places?	YES___ NO___
Do I hear better when only one person speaks?	YES___ NO___
Do I have trouble hearing on the telephone?	YES___ NO___
Do I have a constant ringing or buzzing in my ears?	YES___ NO___
Do I often miss hearing the doorbell or a knock on the door?	YES___ NO___
Do I hear the turn signal in my car?	YES___ NO___
Does my family complain that I play the TV or radio too loud?	YES___ NO___
Do people complain that I don't pay attention to what they say?	YES___ NO___
Have I often been around loud noise?	YES___ NO___
Do members of my family have hearing problems?	YES___ NO___

How did you do? If you answered YES to any of the questions, you may have a hearing loss. Schedule a hearing evaluation to find out for sure.

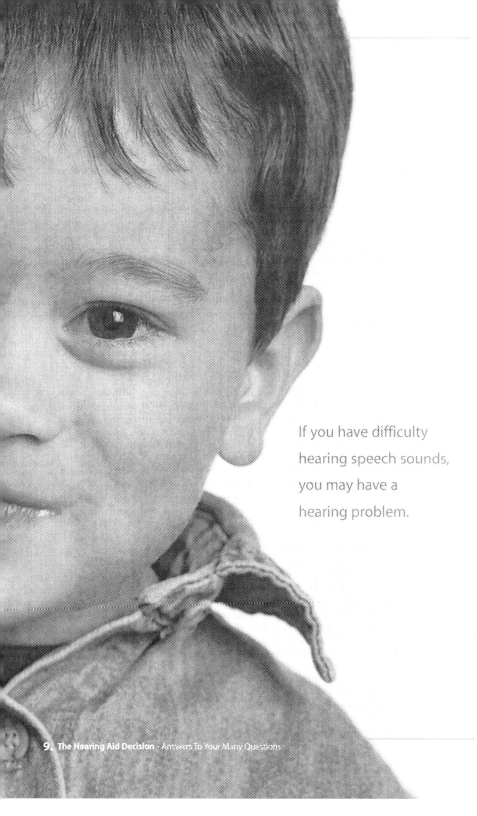

If you have difficulty
hearing speech sounds,
you may have a
hearing problem.

Chapter 2

How's My Hearing?

1. *What is hearing?*

Hearing is about sound. There are a range of sounds – those we use to communicate (speech) and those that are not part of our human communication. The sounds we use to communicate are the speech sounds of our language. If you have difficulty hearing speech sounds, you may have a hearing problem.

There are two technical aspects of sound you should understand. One is the pitch (or frequency) and the other is intensity (or loudness). When hearing is tested, the loudness levels necessary to hear a range of frequencies are evaluated. The test determines how loud the sounds have to be for you to hear them. The information is recorded on a chart called an audiogram. Your hearing health provider will show you the audiogram when explaining the results of your hearing evaluation. (See Audiogram Chart below).

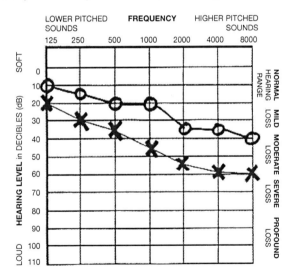

The audiogram contains different symbols: The O's represent the hearing levels in the right ear. The X's represent the hearing levels in the left ear. The numbers at the top of the graph represent the pitches or frequencies; usually tested from 250 Hz (cycles per second) to 8000 Hz.

The numbers on the left side of the graph represent how hearing is measured in terms of loudness or intensity. The greater the number of decibels, the louder the sound has to be before you can hear it. A general classification follows:

If your hearing is between:

0-25 decibels	your hearing is normal
25-40 decibels	is "mild" hearing loss
40-70 decibels	is "moderate" hearing loss
70-90 decibels	is "severe" hearing loss
Greater than 90 decibels	is "profound" hearing loss

The designation of a "mild" hearing loss may give a sense that there isn't a significant hearing problem. It is important to consider to what extent a hearing loss causes problems in everyday communication situations. Even a "mild" hearing loss can cause difficulty and affect the ability to communicate easily. It also is important to note that children in an educational setting may have some difficulty with hearing levels as low as 15 or 20 decibels.

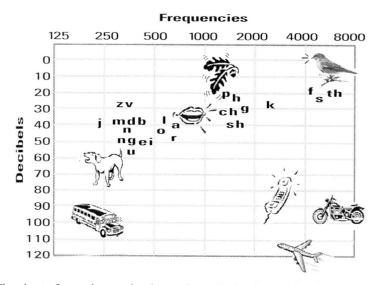

The chart of speech sounds, above, shows the loudness of both environmental and speech sounds. Relate the chart to your personal audiogram. You will observe how loud some noises can be: a motorcycle, a bus, a jet airplane and birds chirping. This helps to reiterate the need for appropriate ear protection for the LOUD noises.

2. *Is hearing loss a common problem?*

Recent surveys (MarkeTrak VII, 2005) have identified that 31.5 million people in the United States report a hearing problem. Approximately 30% of people over the age of 65 have a hearing loss. If you have a hearing problem, you are not alone.

The chart below displays the percentage of people with hearing loss by age group. As you can see, the incidence of hearing loss increases as we grow older but hearing loss affects people of all age groups.

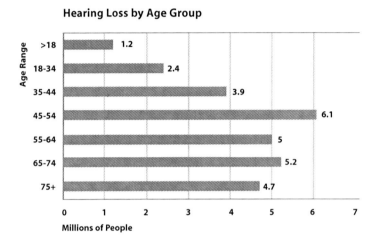

Hearing Loss by Age Group

3. *What causes hearing loss?*

While there are various causes of hearing loss, the two major factors are aging (presbycusis) and noise exposure. Other factors include certain drugs, heredity, colds and other illnesses (especially those with high fever). Your hearing health care provider can discuss causes with you.

4. *What other problems may emerge as a result of hearing loss?*

People may experience fear, anger, embarrassment or anxiety because of the effect hearing loss has on their lives. Some individuals feel isolated from family and friends or left out of the mainstream because of the loss. Some behaviors that appear to be "confusion" due to senility may actually be caused by hearing loss. Hearing loss is a family problem but by working together, we can help those with loss become part of the everyday hearing world.

5. *What is the difference between deafness and hearing impairment?*

These terms describe different degrees of hearing problems. Hearing impairment can describe any amount of hearing loss. Usually, terms such as mild, moderate, severe or profound will indicate the severity of the hearing loss. Deafness refers to profound or total loss of hearing in which hearing aids may be of no help.

6. *What are the types of hearing loss?*

Generally we refer to three categories of hearing loss:

SENSORINEURAL: This is the most common type of hearing loss for adults. Some causes are growing older, high fever illnesses, drugs, noise exposure and heredity. "Nerve deafness" is a term that has been used to refer to a sensorineural hearing loss.

CONDUCTIVE: This type of loss occurs when speech and other sounds cannot pass through the outer and middle ear to the hearing nerve. Causes of a conductive loss may include middle ear infections, excess ear wax in the ear canals, and various diseases. Conductive hearing losses can often be corrected without hearing aids.

MIXED: It is possible for individuals to have both a sensorineural and a conductive loss.

Identifying the type of hearing loss is necessary in order to determine the appropriate approach for treating it.

7. *How does hearing loss impact everyday conversations?*

If your loss is:

MILD: You can hear most conversations but it may seem that some people mumble, especially if there are background noises.

MODERATE: You may need to strain to hear.

SEVERE: You may be unable to hear adequately in most conversations.

PROFOUND: You probably hear nothing unless someone shouts.

8. *What sounds would I have trouble hearing if I have high frequency hearing loss?*

You could have difficulty hearing the speech sounds made by the letters (s), (sh), (ch), (f), (t), (h), (p) and (th) [as in thumb]. For example, you might not be able to distinguish between the words "fifty" or "sixty". The (f) and the (s) are high frequency sounds.

If you have high frequency hearing loss, you may say, "I can hear but cannot understand all of the words." You could also have difficulty hearing birds singing or young children (because these sounds are higher frequencies).

9. *What sounds would I have trouble hearing if I have low frequency hearing loss?*

You might have trouble hearing vowel sounds such as (a), (e), (i), (o) and (u). Conversations may sound muffled unless people are speaking loudly.

10. *Why can I hear men's voices better than the voices of women or young children?*

Men's voices are usually lower pitched; women and young children's voices are usually high pitched. Many men with hearing loss have diminished high frequency hearing, which explains why they may say their wives (or other women) just aren't speaking clearly. They may also have trouble hearing children.

11. *Why do men seem to have more hearing problems than women?*

Men are more likely to be exposed to loud noise from military service, hunting, power mowers and chain saws. However, this appears to be changing in our society through more diversity of employment.

12. *How do I hear sounds and speech?*

The diagram below illustrates the three main parts of the ear:

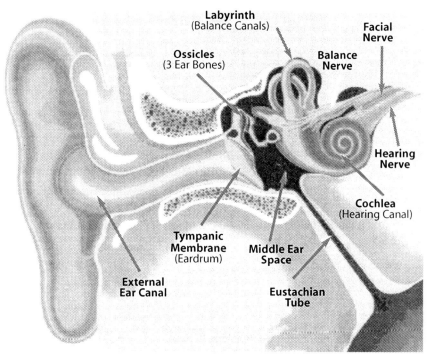

Courtesy of Starkey Laboratories

The outer ear is the part of the ear we can see as well as the ear canal that goes to the eardrum (tympanic membrane). This outer portion of the ear collects the sounds of speech and funnels them to the eardrum.

The middle ear is an air-filled cavity behind the eardrum. As the eardrum vibrates, the vibrations are transferred through three little bones - the hammer, anvil and stirrup (ossicles) - to the inner ear.

The ossicles transfer the mechanical sound through the oval window (the beginning of the inner ear) into the sensorineural part of the ear. The inner ear is where mechanical sounds are converted into nerve impulses which are then transmitted to the brain.

Conductive losses which we mentioned in Question #6 occur in the outer and middle ear. Sensorineural hearing losses occur in the inner ear and the nerve pathway to the brain.

13. *Are certain frequencies more important for hearing speech than others?*

All of the frequencies shown on the audiogram are important, however, because high frequency hearing loss is common in adults this can cause intelligibility problems.

14. *How loud is normal, everyday speech?*

Normal conversational speech is about 50-60 dB.

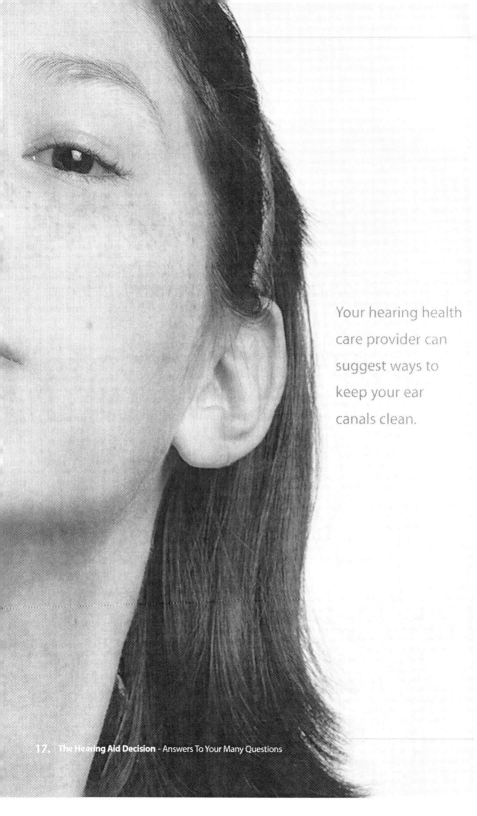

Your hearing health care provider can suggest ways to keep your ear canals clean.

Chapter 3
Caring For Your Ears

1. *Why is there wax in my ears?*

Cerumen (ear wax) in the ear is normal. The ear wax lubricates the skin in the ear canal, kills bacteria and helps keep the ear canal from becoming too dry and itchy. Too much wax, however, can block sound and cause conductive hearing loss.

2. *Should I use a cotton-tipped swab or other items to remove wax from my ears?*

Using these items to remove wax can cause infections and discomfort in the ear canal. Sticks with cotton tips may be soft, but the cotton strands can become stuck in ear wax. As you continue to try to remove the wax, you may actually push the wax farther down into the ear canal. Your hearing health care provider can suggest ways to keep your canals clean (various ear drops may be available for you). If your ears feel plugged or your hearing gets worse you should see your hearing health care provider. Ask your physician to determine if you have excessive wax in your ears at your next physical examination.

3. *Will using hearing aids cause more ear wax?*

In-the-ear hearing aids may cause increased ear wax. By following appropriate suggestions for ear hygiene, problems due to excessive ear wax can be reduced. Routinely cleaning your hearing aids reduces ear wax getting into the aids.

4. *What should I do about itching in my ear?*

If you have chronic itching in the ear canal, schedule an appointment with your hearing health care provider who can suggest ways to reduce the itching or refer you to your physician for a medical assessment.

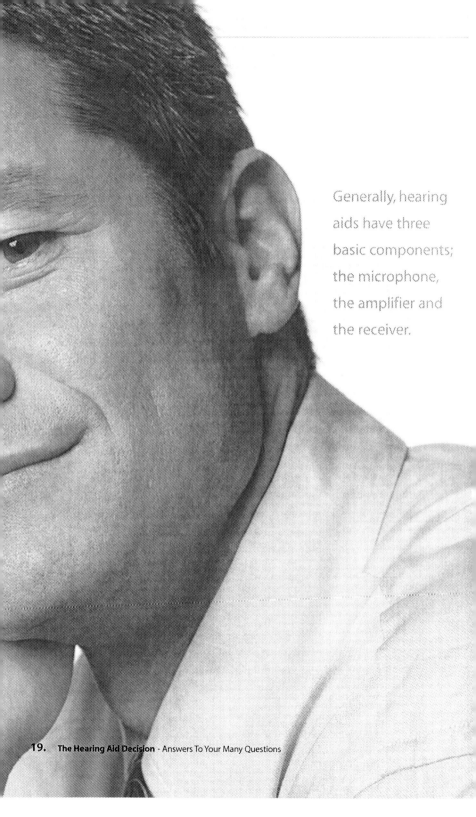

Generally, hearing aids have three basic components; the microphone, the amplifier and the receiver.

Chapter 4

Hearing Aid Basics

1. *What is a hearing aid?*

Hearing aids are compact, high tech, electronic sound amplification systems encased in plastic. They amplify sounds so the listener can hear better. For people with severe hearing loss, hearing aids can help them hear sirens, traffic and noises for a safer environment.

2. *What are the major parts of hearing aids and what do they do?*

Generally, hearing aids have three basic components; the microphone, the amplifier and the receiver.

- The microphone receives sound and converts it into an electrical signal.
- The amplifier increases the power of the signal and sends it to the receiver.
- The receiver converts the electronic signal back to speech sounds, which are transmitted to your ears.

3. *What is an ear mold?*

For people who choose "behind-the-ear" (BTE) hearing aids, ear molds are necessary so that the sound can be delivered via tubing to the ear. The ear mold is usually a custom fitted ear piece that is the exact shape of the bowl part of your outer ear and ear canal. Impressions are taken for the ear molds. There are BTE aids that can now be worn without earmolds. Ask your provider about this option.

4. *What are the various designs or types of hearing aids?*

There are several different designs and sizes of hearing aids. These include:

• **Completely-in-the-Canal (CICs):**
This design fits down into the ear canal
and is not very visible. With this small size,
changing the batteries and placement in
the ear may be difficult without good
manual dexterity.

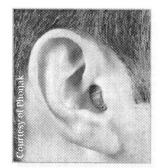

CIC

• **In-the-Canal (ITCs):** These aids are
somewhat larger than the CICs but still are
relatively small. They are easier to manipulate than the smaller CIC size.

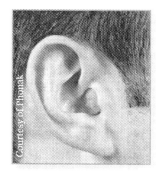

ITC

• **Half Shell:** The Half Shell size is between the ITC and the Full Shell aids. They
often are a compromise for people who don't want the smallest or the largest aids.

• **In-the-Ear (Full Shell or ITEs):** These aids
are larger and fit in the bowl in you outer ear
which leads to your ear canal. Most people
are able to manipulate the volume control,
batteries, and placement more easily with
the larger size, however, this style is more
visible.

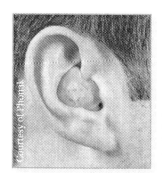

*Full
Shell
or
ITE*

• **Behind-the-Ear (BTEs):** These aids fit behind and over the ear. A plastic tube connects the hearing aids to the earmolds that fits into the ear canals. Young children are often fit with this type of aid since, as the ear changes, only new earmolds, rather than new aids are required. Some individuals with severe and profound losses may do better with BTE aids.

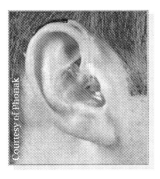

BTE

• **CROS, Bi-CROS, and Multi-CROS** hearing aids are used specifically when the hearing in one ear is much worse or a total loss compared to the other ear. In this situation, a microphone is placed on the more impaired ear and held in place by a Behind-the-Ear device. Sound is transmitted to the hearing aids in the better ear either by a wire that goes behind the head or by a wireless system. The hearing aid in the better ear picks up the sounds from the microphone in the more impaired ear, then transmits the sounds into the hearing aid in the less impaired ear. (Check with your provider about technology advances).

• **Totally Open Canal, Open Fit and Open Ear:** These small on-the-ear hearing aids may be appropriate for some hearing losses. Typical candidates are people who have normal or near normal hearing in the low and mid-pitch range but sensorineural hearing loss in the high pitch range. Each open hearing aid has its own criteria for candidacy. These hearing aids may have a speaker that is seated in the ear canal or a small, clear thin tube that fits into the ear canal. One benefit of open hearing aids is that they make your own voice seem more natural and eliminates that "plugged up" feeling. These hearing aids are cosmetically appealing because of their small size.

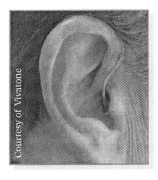
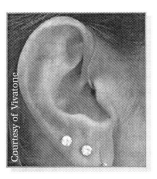

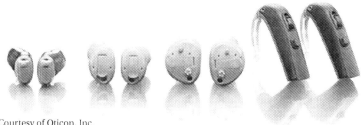

Courtesy of Oticon, Inc.

There are various designs and options with most of the above aids. You can obtain information from your hearing health care provider.

5. *What are programmable hearing aids?*

Programmable aids represent some of the latest technological advances in amplification. These hearing instruments have several programming parameters which can be adjusted on a computer and set for different listening situations. For example, one program may be set for a quiet situation, a second program for listening in noise, and a third for listening to music. Changing programs may be done by pushing a button on the hearing aids or, in some cases, optional remote controls are available. These programmable hearing aids typically use digital technology which makes auditory signals more precise. Most hearing aids purchased today contain digital technology.

With programmable hearing aids it is possible to "test drive" the technology in the provider's office before making a purchase.

Continuing research and development in hearing aid technology, as in other computer and electronic instrumentation, will result in the continuing development of improved hearing instruments.

6. *What does the term "fit" mean when someone speaks about the fit or fitting of hearing aids?*

The term "fit" is broadly used to refer to placing the hearing aids in the ear, making all necessary adjustments, and programming the aids (if applicable) to the satisfaction of the client.

7. *Do hearing aids come in different colors?*

The shells of hearing aids come in a variety of colors and skin tones. Some common skin tone colors are pink, beige, tan, dark brown and light brown. Young children often choose a color for their hearing aids.

8. *Why do my hearing aids whistle?*

The whistle (also called feedback) is due to sound from the hearing aids being re-amplified. Whistling can happen if:

- The ear mold does not fit properly. If this is the problem, the ear mold will need to be remade.

- There is excessive wax in the ear canal.

- The hearing aids or earmolds are cracked or not seated in your ear properly or snugly.

- You cup your hand around your ear or improperly place a telephone receiver up to your ear.

- The volume of the hearing aids is turned up too loud.

- The ear canal moves when you chew or pull on your earlobe. The seal between the hearing aid and the ear canal is not a good fit.

9. *What causes background noise?*

Background noises are present in the environment and affect people who hear normally as well as hearing aid users. Background noises you hear through the hearing aids are usually caused by excessive low frequency sounds such as road noise, fans, people talking and a host of other factors. If your hearing aids aren't working properly, the result can be unwanted background noise. Various types of hearing aids and adjustment options can reduce this particular problem.

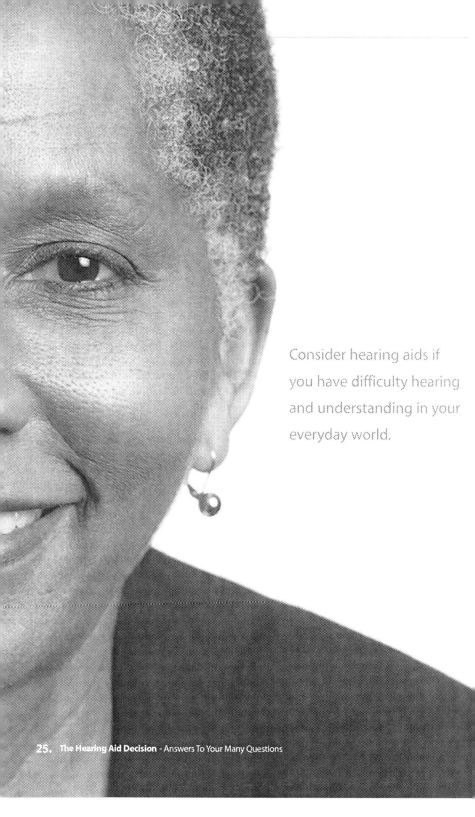

Consider hearing aids if
you have difficulty hearing
and understanding in your
everyday world.

Chapter 5
The Hearing Aid Decision

1. *How significant should my hearing loss be before I consider hearing aids?*

Consider hearing aids if you have difficulty hearing and understanding in your everyday world. Look at the results of your Self Test and also ask for input from your family and others.

2. *What are some of the possible benefits of using hearing aids?*

• Your hearing will be enhanced so you can hear and understand speech more easily.

• You will be more comfortable (less embarrassed) in social situations.

• You will strain less when listening to other people.

• Conversations on the telephone will be easier to understand.

• You will be able to hear and understand conversations better when there is background noise.

• You will be able to better understand speech in many social situations.

• Your own voice will sound more natural.

• You may have better job opportunities if you are employed or seeking employment.

• You will be able to better appreciate music.

• Your hearing loss may be less apparent to others.

• Speech may sound more natural to you.

3. *What are some things that my hearing aids may not do?*

• Hearing aids may not completely restore your hearing to its pre-loss level, but you should hear better.

• Hearing aids may not remove all background noise; however, newer technology has greatly reduced this problem.

• Hearing aids cannot prevent hearing from decreasing over time.

• Hearing aids cannot cure the physical hearing loss, but they can help you hear and better communicate.

4. *What types of hearing losses can hearing aids help?*

Hearing aids can help enhance the hearing of people with either conductive or sensorineural hearing losses.

5. *Can I use someone else's hearing aids?*

Your hearing loss is unique to you so you need hearing aids that are specifically selected for your loss. Your hearing health care provider can suggest the appropriate hearing aids for your situation.

6. *Will hearing aids make my hearing worse or prevent it from decreasing?*

Properly fitted hearing aids should not make your hearing worse or prevent it from decreasing. If you feel that your hearing is deteriorating however, you should see your hearing health care provider. Generally, a hearing loss due to aging occurs slowly over the years. Annual hearing checks are advisable to track your hearing.

7. *Will hearing aids help me hear better in noisy places?*

Correctly selected and fitted hearing aids should help you understand speech better in noisy situations. How well they help depends on the type and loudness of the noise and the degree of your hearing loss. If the aids do not seem to help, ask your provider if they can be adjusted to improve your understanding when there is background noise. Keep in mind that people with normal hearing have difficulty in extremely noise settings, too. (Observe how many people seem to shout at each other in a noisy restaurant.)

8. *Can hearing aids help make me feel more relaxed?*

If you have a hearing problem, listening can be hard work. Many hearing aid users report that they feel more relaxed when using hearing aids. They tend to feel less frustration or fear of not hearing what is said. At the end of the day, the hearing aid user may feel less tired and more relaxed.

9. *Will hearing aids make my ear feel plugged?*

Hearing aids may make you ear feel plugged, and as a new user, it may take some time to adjust to the fact that something is in your ear. Your voice may sound funny to you at first. Hearing aids and ear molds can be made with various types of vents which allow air to circulate between the outer part of the hearing aids and the space inside the ear canal facing the eardrum. This helps to reduce the plugged feeling. If you feel a hollow or barrel type of sensation, your hearing health care provider can make various adjustments to reduce this feeling. Remember that it may take a little time to adjust to your new hearing aids.

10. *Am I too old to wear hearing aids?*

Using hearing aids is not an age thing. Any person who can be helped by hearing aids should use hearing aids. Your ears can be younger or older than your age.

11. *Will one type of hearing aid work for every hearing loss?*

No. There is not one hearing aid that will work for all hearing losses. Your hearing health care provider will evaluate all available options to help you make the best choice for your lifestyle.

12. *Loud sounds bother me. Will hearing aids make sounds too loud?*

Hearing aids use circuits that can prevent sounds (such as shouting children or the banging of pots and pans) from being too loud. Your hearing evaluation will determine the kinds of adjustments that may be necessary for your new hearing aids to prevent or reduce this problem. Remember to remove your aids when mowing lawns or using chain saws.

13. *Can I use hearing aids with the telephone?*

In most instances, you can use your aids with the telephone. If your hearing aids whistle or speech is not clear, you may select hearing aids with a telecoil (t-coil) option. With this set up, you can easily switch to the t-coil. Your provider will help determine the best way to use the telephone with your hearing aids

14. *Why do some people who need hearing aids refuse to purchase them?*

- Not psychologically ready.
- Unaware of the extent of their hearing loss since the loss occurred gradually.
- A feeling that hearing aids carry a stigma of "old age".
- Don't think hearing aids can help them.
- Think hearing aids are too expensive.

15. *Why do some people refuse to wear hearing aids after they purchase them?*

- Lack of personal motivation.
- Did not want the aids but purchased them due to pressure from family.
- Embarrassed to wear hearing aids.
- Too much trouble to maintain their aids on daily basis.
- Expectation levels are not being met.
- Need two aids but purchased only one.
- Aids aren't really helping.
- Background noise is too bothersome.

- Aids are uncomfortable.
- Unwilling to ask for help from the provider if aids are not fit or working properly.
- May not have received sufficient orientation after the purchase.

Your hearing health care provider can help you determine and overcome the problems listed above or any problems that exist for you. Do not hesitate to ask for help. Take advantage of the one, two or three month adjustment period provided by the manufacturer.

Notes:

There are several types
of providers who
dispense hearing aids.

Chapter 6
Now What?

1. *Who sells or dispenses hearing aids?*

There are several types of providers who dispense hearing aids. Regardless of the provider, consumers need to make sure the individual possesses the appropriate credentials. There are both national and state requirements for licensure or certification. You can contact your State Board of Regulatory Agencies to determine whether your provider is appropriately credentialed.

Providers may include the following:

Audiologists: Certified by the American Speech-Language-Hearing Association (CCC-A) and/or by state regulatory agencies. Some may be Fellows or Board Certified by the American Academy of Audiology. The minimum degree nationally is a Master's Degree; many audiologists now earn a Doctor of Audiology degree (Au.D.). Audiologists, in addition to dispensing hearing aids, specialize in the diagnostic and rehabilitative aspects of hearing and balance.

Hearing Aid Dispensers: Certified (BC-HIS) by the National Board for Certification in Hearing Instrument Sciences (NBC-HIS). They may also need to be accredited by a state regulatory agency. BCHIS individuals emphasize hearing evaluation, hearing aid selection and fitting.

In this book, we use the terms Hearing Health Care Provider, Hearing Aid Provider or just Provider.

2. *How should I choose my hearing aid provider?*

- Find a provider with an established, conveniently located office with easy parking.

- Make sure the provider is available to provide service when it is convenient for you.

- Make sure providers have appropriate credentials.

- Make sure the provider appears to be sensitive to your needs.

3. *What are the steps involved in buying hearing aids?*

- Have your hearing evaluated and discuss the findings and recommendations with your provider.

- Get a second hearing test and opinion if you feel it is necessary.

- See a physician as necessary.

- Select your hearing aid(s). Ask whether you have an adjustment period (often referred to as trial period) with the hearing aids. Most providers offer 30 days or more. Most will refund your money if you are not pleased with the performance of the aids. Some may charge a minimal fee for the return of the hearing aids.

- Follow-up as necessary for proper fit and performance.

4. *Can I have my hearing tested at home?*

Some hearing aid providers will make house calls. A complete hearing evaluation, however, should be done in a hearing health care provider's office. Home visits are usually reserved for people with significant mobility or transportation issues.

5. *Do I need to see a medical doctor before I purchase hearing aids?*

You should see a physician if you have any of these problems:

- A visible or traumatic deformity or injury to the ear.
- Drainage from the ear within the previous 90 days.
- Acute or chronic dizziness.
- A sudden or rapidly progressing hearing loss within the past 90 days.
- A hearing loss in only one ear of sudden or recent onset.
- A conductive type hearing loss.
- Visible evidence of ear wax or a foreign body in the ear canal.
- Pain or discomfort in the ears.

The Food and Drug Administration (FDA) advocates that adults and children should have a medical evaluation prior to purchasing hearing aids. The physician can determine if any medical problems exist that are related to your hearing problem. Your physician will provide you with a medical clearance for hearing aids. Adults, however, may choose not to see a physician and waive this requirement by signing a medical waiver.

6. *What are some factors to consider in selecting hearing aids?*

The decision for the type of hearing aids you purchase depends on the degree of your hearing loss, the anatomy of your outer ear and ear canal, your personal needs and your ability to use a specific type of aid. Discuss the questions below with your provider to help you select the aids that will work best for you:

- What benefits can I expect?
- Will the hearing aids provide me with optimum benefits for my needs?
- What do hearing aids cost?
- What other costs may be included?
- Are the hearing aids easy to manipulate? They should be easy to insert into the ears, change the batteries and adjust the volume controls.
- How easy is it to get service and adjustments when I need them?
- What is the warranty period? How much does it cost and how long is it valid?
- How easily can the aids be inserted and removed?
- How easily can the controls on the aids be adjusted?
- Do hearing aids come with special options to meet my specific needs?
- Can the hearing aids be adjusted if my hearing loss changes?
- Do the hearing aids have the options (telecoil, adjustable volume control, on-off switch, tone control, etc.) I need?
- Are the hearing aids comfortable?
- Is the cost a factor in your decision?
- Is the cosmetic appearance acceptable?

All of these factors should be considered. If you purchase aids solely on the basis of cosmetic appeal, you may get expensive aids that may be difficult for you to manage. If you get the lowest cost aids, they may not be ideal for your situation.

There are no consumer guides to show which specific aids are best for YOU, however, your provider can help you choose the brand and type of hearing aids that should produce the best results. That is why selecting your provider is such an important decision.

7. *Do I need one or two aids?*

Our two ears help us hear at work, at school, outdoors, in our recreational activities, and when we watch television and listen to the radio. Having two ears helps us localize where sound and speech come from and helps us to hear more clearly. There are exceptions in where one ear may have a profound loss and an aid just won't work well. It is possible that, after the adjustment period, you find that one aid may be more appropriate for you.

8. *Should I buy the smallest aids available?*

Often, people want to purchase the smallest amplification devices available because they are less noticeable. While cosmetics are important, your major concern should be selecting the hearing aids that help you best. For some, the best just might be the smallest and least visible.

Notes:

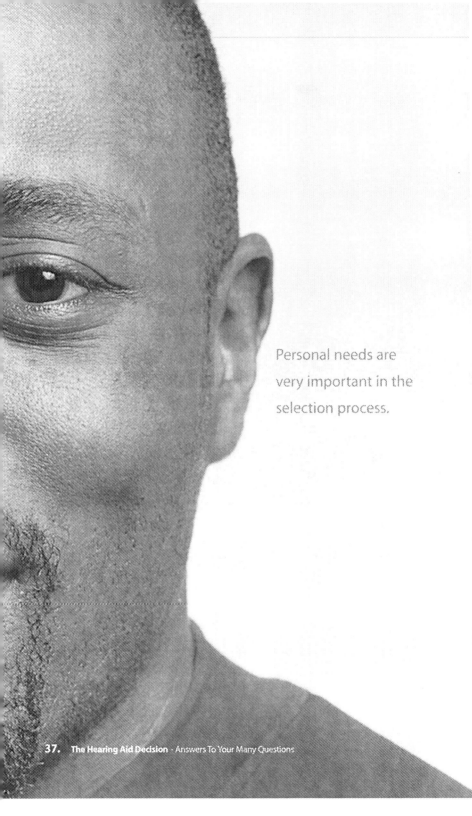

Personal needs are
very important in the
selection process.

Chapter 7

Purchasing Your Hearing Aid

1. *How much do hearing aids cost?*

The cost of hearing aids often includes your hearing evaluation, the hearing aids and warranty guarantees. Ask your provider about hearing aid options in the price range that best meets your needs. The type of hearing system you and your hearing healthcare provider select should be based on your hearing needs.

As noted in Chapter 4, there are open ear aids, BTE, ITE, ITC, and CIC types. Usually the smaller aids are more expensive due to the need for miniature circuitry.

Most hearing aids manufactured today use digital technology and are pro-grammable, however, non-digital hearing aids are still available from some manufacturers.

Personal needs are very important in the selection process. For example, a person living alone with less need for communication may be able to get along with aids that are less expensive. Compare this with someone such as a physician or sales person who has considerable contact with others and needs to hear conversations accurately.

It is a good idea to discuss your personal needs with your hearing health care provider and your family.

Some advertising which states claims of pricing or benefits may be exaggerated. The value of your hearing aids can be based on how they improve the quality of your life.

2. *What is the rationale for the pricing of hearing aids?*

There are many factors that contribute to the cost of hearing aids, including:

- Research and development of technologies and rapid change in technologies.
- The limited number of units sold nationally.
- High level of professional services involved in dispensing and servicing.
- Warranty costs.
- Marketing costs.
- Costs associated with units returned for credit.

3. *Will my health insurance pay for hearing aids?*

Many insurance programs cover the cost of hearing tests but not the cost of hearing aids. Ask your health insurance representative.

4. *Does Medicare cover the cost of hearing aids?*

Medicare does not pay for the hearing tests used in the selection and fitting of hearing aids nor does it pay for hearing aids. Laws vary from state to state though, so please check the current guidelines.

5. *Are there organizations that can help cover the cost of my hearing aids?*

If the cost of hearing aids is what stands between you and better hearing, there are organizations that may be able to help you. Two organizations that serve nationally are:

- **HearNow, Starkey Laboratories**
  6700 Washington Ave, Eden Prairie, MN 33025, 800-769-2799
- **Friends of Man**
  P.O. Box 937, Littleton CO 80120, 303-798-2342 • www.friendsofman.org

There are also various local civic and religious organizations that provide assistance. Check with your provider about help available in your area.

6. *Should I use a credit card to pay for the aids?*

This, of course, is a matter of choice. Charging the hearing aids to a credit card, however, can give you additional consumer protection should you not receive the products or services for which you paid. Within limits, the credit card company can help assure that you get the products and services you were promised. If you dispute any aspect of the sale, quality or delivery of the hearing aids or their performance, the credit card company may withhold payment until the dispute is settled. Prior to making your payment decision, you may wish to ask if there is a discount for cash.

7. *Can I get the hearing aids the same day I order them?*

Often you can get open canal or BTE aids the same day. The aids can be adjusted to fit your hearing loss and universal ear molds (or stock molds) can often be used to fit in your ear. If you have a moderate or severe hearing loss, you may need to have hearing aids and ear molds ordered for you.

Most in-the-ear (ITE) hearing aids must be specifically manufactured for your ear. Same day delivery of these custom made aids is not generally possible.

8. *What are the benefits and pitfalls of ordering aids through the mail or online?*

Mail order hearing aids are usually less expensive than those you purchase from a hearing aid provider, however, the aids usually are generic - one type fits all - and, they may not be the right aids for you. Generic aids may amplify sounds that you do not need. Hearing aids will work better for you if selected and fit by your provider for your specific level of hearing loss. It is important to consult a professional to work directly with you to more effectively fit and service the aids.

There are some providers who will allow you to order hearing aids through the Internet or mail and who will then fit you for a fee and provide all follow-up. You may save money ordering by mail or online but you will lose the personalized service you receive from a local provider.

You can prolong
the life of your
hearing aids by
taking care of
them according
to the manufacturer's
instructions.

Chapter 8

Hearing Aid Care And Maintenance

1. *What is the average lifespan of hearing aids?*

The average lifespan, as a general guideline, ranges from three to five years for ITE aids and five to seven years for BTE aids. How long they last depends on their use and care, how the technology meets your continuing needs and changes which may occur in your hearing. You can prolong the life of your hearing aids by taking care of them according to the manufacturer's instructions. It is also a good idea to have your provider check and clean them periodically, especially if your ears produce a considerable amount of wax. Improper care and environmental pollutants can reduce the life of hearing aids.

2. *How long do hearing aid batteries last?*

The life of hearing aid batteries depends on the power of the aids and how many hours per day you use the aids. It also depends on the type of battery you use. Generally, the smaller the battery, the shorter the battery life. Your hearing aid provider can give you the manufacturer's estimate about the length of time the batteries will last. Smaller batteries may last 5-10 days; larger batteries may last two to four weeks. It is a good idea to keep an extra package of batteries with you at all times.

3. *What are the major causes of hearing aids not functioning properly and what can I do?*

There are a number of reasons your hearing aids may not function properly. Excessive ear wax is a common problem, especially if the aids are not cleaned on a regular basis. Weak or dead batteries may also cause problems and should be replaced regularly. You can do some of your own trouble-shooting if your hearing aids are not working. Before scheduling service, be sure to check the following:

- Is there ear wax in the canal opening of the aids which could block sound?

- Is the battery dead? (You can purchase an inexpensive battery tester.)

- Is the battery placed in the compartment properly?

- Is the hearing aid turned on and the volume adjusted to a comfortable listening level?

- If you have a telecoil, is the switch in the correct position?

- If the hearing aid works intermittently, that is usually a sign that there is an internal problem. If this situation persists, contact your provider.

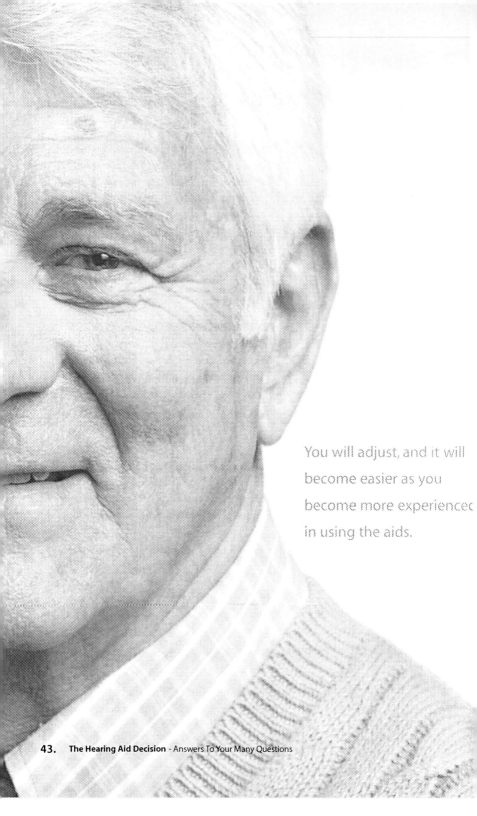

You will adjust, and it will become easier as you become more experienced in using the aids.

Chapter 9
Adjusting To Your New Hearing Aids

1. *How do I learn to use hearing aids?*

Learning to use hearing aids requires some personal motivation. It's not the same as putting on a pair of eyeglasses and walking out of the doctor's office. It is an activity that requires your involvement in each step of the fitting process.

When you are given the hearing aids, your provider will review the information in the user's brochure that comes with the aids and show you how to adjust the volume control and other switches, if applicable. You will also be shown where the volume control should be set, how to insert and remove the aids from your ear and how to change the battery.

For the first week or so, wear the aids around your home to give yourself time to become accustomed to the way they sound. Use the hearing aids when you talk to friends or listen to television. After a few days, you can begin to wear them outside your home. If the aids are uncomfortable, turn them down or off for a period of time. Then turn them on again later. Do not remove them from your ears unless they physically hurt. Give yourself time to get adjusted to how they feel in your ear.

It is important to remember that some individuals adjust quickly to amplification and need little adjustment time. For others, the process takes longer. Keep practicing. Be patient. You will adjust and it will become easier as you become more experienced in using the aids. If you continue to have difficulty, return to your provider so the aids can be checked and adjusted as needed.

2. *Are there some specific things I can do during the adjustment period?*

Yes. When wearing your hearing aids for the first time, you may hear sounds that you have not heard for a long time. Be patient as your brain relearns to use and understand these sounds.

Some people adjust quickly; others need more time. If you are having difficulty adjusting, consider using the activities on the following page.

- Practice putting your hearing aids on and adjusting controls.

- For short periods of time, wear your aids in a quiet room and read aloud to yourself. (Speak clearly. Listen to your own voice.)

- Talk with one person at a time from a distance not greater than six feet.

- Ask the person to speak in a clear, natural voice - not too fast or too slow.

- Watch the speaker all of the time and put together what you see and hear (auditory-visual cues).

- Try to reduce the amount of background noise in all listening situations. Television, air conditioners, dishwashers and other noisy appliances can make communication more difficult.

- Listen to radio or recorded music. Ask a family member to set the volume of the radio or TV so they can hear it comfortably at a distance of six feet.

- Gradually increase the time you wear your hearing aids. Turn them off if they make you tired or nervous. Wear the aids as long as you can comfortably tolerate them.

3. *How do I know if the hearing aids help me?*

After you have used the aids for several days, ask yourself the following questions.

- Can I more easily hear and better understand what I hear?
- Do I understand speech better?
- Do I hear non-speech sounds better?
- Have others told me that I hear better?

In addition, review your Self Test at the front of the book. And last but not least, ask your spouse or significant other. That may be the best test of all!

4. *How do I know if my hearing aids fit properly?*

The hearing aids should fit comfortably and snugly in your ear. A comfortable fit is important because you may be wearing the aids 12-16 hours a day. A snug fit is necessary so you can turn the aids loud enough to help you hear without feedback. Ccorrectly-fitted aids will help you hear and understand speech. The sounds from the aids should be comfortably loud. They should not be distorted. Background noises should not be excessively loud compared to the sounds of conversational speech.

5. *How do I care for my hearing aids?*

DO these things:

- Do clean your aids with a dry cloth every night.
- Do remove the battery or open the battery drawer every night to extend battery life.
- Do remove hearing aids before bathing, showering, shaving or swimming.
- Do keep your hearing aids as dry as possible when engaged in activities that produce perspiration.
- Do remove your aids while fixing your hair or using hairspray.
- To avoid whistling or feedback, turn the hearing aids off when inserting or removing them.

DON'T do these things:

- Don't drop your hearing aids or jar them unnecessarily.
- Don't expose your aids to extreme heat or cold.
- Don't leave your aids where they can be picked up by small children or animals.
- Don't stick pins, paper clips or anything in the hearing aid openings.
- Don't attempt to repair the hearing aids yourself.
- Don't take your hearing aids apart to examine them for any reason. Taking your aids apart will void the manufacturer's warranty.
- Don't allow the hearing aids to become wet, as serious damage may result.

6. *What other things can I do to help improve my hearing?*

Years ago, prior to the significant advances in hearing aid technology, recommendations were sometimes made for procedures referred to as lip reading (speech reading), auditory training, and aural rehabilitation. The belief was that using a multi-sensory approach, i.e., hearing and vision, individuals would be able to communicate more easily than if they were relying only on their hearing. These approaches are used less often today. However, there are some strategies that may help you communicate better.

Controlling or manipulating your listening environment can help. You can do some or all of the following to improve your ability to communicate more easily:

- The speaker and listener should face each other. The use of visual cues to supplement auditory cues may help compensate for "missed" portions of conversation.
- Stand five to 10 feet from the speaker. Don't speak from another room.
- Avoid light directly in the listener's eyes or face. Lighting should be overhead or slightly in front of the speaker.
- Decrease competing background noise when possible. For example, turn off the dishwasher.

The person speaking to you can also contribute to how easily you can communicate with them. The following are conversation tips for those speaking to individuals who have hearing loss:

- Speak normally and pronounce words clearly.
- Rephrase a conversation if the person has difficulty understanding it.
- Do not cover your mouth or turn away when speaking.
- Do not assume that if a person is wearing hearing aids you should talk louder.
- Do not assume that hearing aids have restored the individual's hearing to "normal."
- The more you talk with a person with hearing loss, the easier it will become for the listener to understand you.

7. *How do I know if my hearing aids fit properly?*

This complaint is most often voiced when someone does not want the hearing aids or when the aids are not correctly selected or adjusted for the hearing loss. You should discuss this problem with your hearing aid provider. It is important for you to work closely with your provider. Most people are able to adjust to their aids, especially after they realize the benefits of hearing and understanding. Patience is a virtue, especially for new hearing aid users.

Remember, if all else fails, you are in an adjustment period and can return the aids for credit or you can try another type.

Notes:

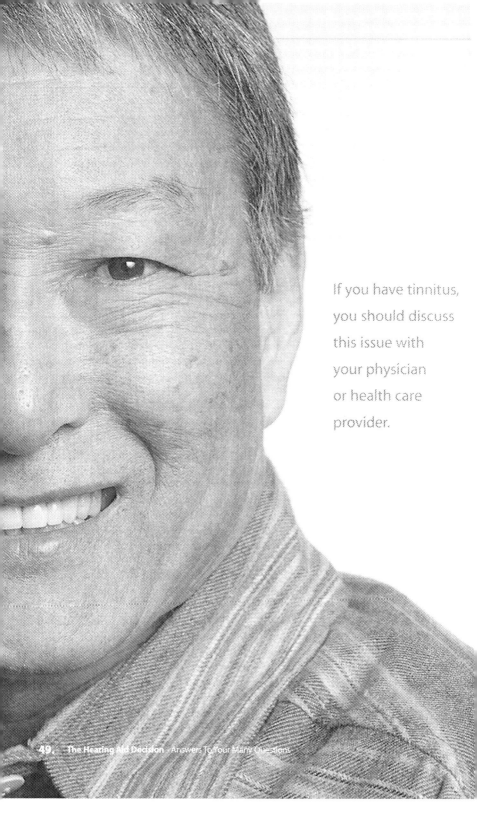

If you have tinnitus,
you should discuss
this issue with
your physician
or health care
provider.

Chapter 10
About That Ringing And Buzzing In My Ears (Tinnitus)

1. *What is tinnitus?*

Tinnitus often is described as a high pitch ringing, buzzing, rushing stream and hissing noise, but is actually defined as the "perception of sound in the absence of environmental noise." (Sullivan, M., Katon, M, Dobie W., et al. Disabling tinnitus-association with affective disorders. Gen Hosp Psychiatry, 1988, 10:258-291). It can be continuous or intermittent. Tinnitus may be heard in one or both ears.

2. *What causes tinnitus?*

Exact causes are not always known as many factors are associated with tinnitus. It is often found in people with hearing loss and is considered a symptom rather than a disease. Some contributing factors may include:

- Aging
- Noise-induced damage
- Ototoxic drugs
- Stress
- High blood pressure
- Aspirin

There may be other causes. If you have tinnitus, you should discuss this issue with your physician or healthcare provider.

Tinnitus can become both a nuisance and a frustration for you. Take a moment to complete the **Tinnitus Questionnaire.** Your answers may help you describe the problem to your physician or healthcare provider so he or she can identify medical treatment to eliminate or reduce the problem. If there is no medical treatment available, you can then discuss with your healthcare provider other options to minimize the problem. Although tinnitus may bothersome to some people others find that it does not affect their lives.

Tinnitus Questionnaire

A. Is the tinnitus constant _____ or intermittent _____?

B. Is the tinnitus in one ear_____ or both ears_____?

C. Circle the words that best describe the sound of the tinnitus:

- ringing   • hissing   • popping   • roaring

- buzzing   • pulsing   • wind   • insects

- other_____

D. Is the tinnitus...

- Masked by environmental sounds?   YES___ NO___
- Interfering with sleep?   YES___ NO___
- Aggravated by any of the following stimuli?
  - noise   YES___ NO___
  - caffeine   YES___ NO___
  - alcohol   YES___ NO___
  - other_____

- Interfering with daily activities?   YES___ NO___
- Handicapping you in any way?   YES___ NO___
- Interfering with family relationships?   YES___ NO___

E. Circle how you would rate the severity of the problem.

- mild

- moderate

- severe

The following factors may contribute or aggravate tinnitus:

- Excess ear wax.
- Hypertension and stress.
- Exposure to loud noises.
- Temporomandibular joint problems.
- Use of quinine, aspirin, anti-inflammatory and other drugs.
- Use of caffeinated and alcoholic drinks.

3. *How is tinnitus treated?*

Exact causes are not always known as many factors are associated with tinnitus. It is often found in people with hearing loss and is considered a symptom rather than a disease.

• To mask out tinnitus, use a recording of pleasant background noise or white noise. Some individuals who have difficulty falling asleep have used this approach. Electronic and record stores may have CDs or tapes.

• Commercial tinnitus maskers worn in the ears, like BTE hearing aids, have been useful for some persons as the maskers "drown out" the tinnitus.

• Relaxation techniques may help to minimize the bothersome effects of tinnitus. Combined with biofeedback, this approach has been beneficial for some with long term tinnitus.

• Certain herbs and medications have been used. Check with your physician regarding this matter.

Continuing research is being done by the American Tinnitus Association (ATA) and others. For years, there has been little interest in tinnitus research but now that seems to be changing. One such study reported by Newman (2006) provides an example of recent research. A new therapy originated in Australia, called Neuromonics, uses a pleasant acoustic signal (embedded in music) presented through earphones at a comfortable listening level. Treatment lasts about six months, and follow up can be done on a weekly or monthly basis. Contact the ATA for additional information. (We recommend a subscription to the ATA Journal to keep informed.)

Although there is not yet a cure, some procedures may help you tolerate tinnitus. Remember that procedures may not work the same way for everyone. Also, be aware that hearing aids have helped some by making environmental sounds and speech louder than the tinnitus.

If you would like more information, contact your hearing health care provider.

Newman, Craig. Roadmap to a Cure: Determining Benefits of Treatment, Journal American Tinnitus Association, 31(4), December 2006, pp 7-9.

Hearing aids are not only a financial investment, but an investment in your health and quality of life.

Chapter 11

Conclusion

The goal of this publication was to inform consumers of the many things they need to be aware of when confronted with the hearing aid decision. We may not have answered all of your questions, but we hope we have provided you with a better understanding of what is involved with your hearing aid purchase, such as whether you actually need an aid, what kind of aid you need, whether you should purchase one aid or two and where to buy the aids. If so, your efforts will result in better hearing.

Hearing aids are not only a financial investment, but an investment in your health and quality of life. There simply are not many things we can do in this society without the ability to speak, to hear and to understand what we hear.

If you have made the hearing aid decision and purchased new hearing aids, we suggest that you retake **My Self Test**, initially presented at the beginning of the book, to see how your responses have changed.

My Self Test

Do I often miss what I want to hear?	YES___ NO___
Do I frequently ask people to repeat themselves?	YES___ NO___
Do I think most people mumble?	YES___ NO___
Do I strain to hear what others are saying?	YES___ NO___
Do I often misunderstand what people say?	YES___ NO___
Do I hear speech sounds, but not understand all of the words?	YES___ NO___
Do I avoid social activities because of my hearing?	YES___ NO___
Do I have trouble understanding people in noisy places?	YES___ NO___
Do I hear better when only one person speaks?	YES___ NO___
Do I have trouble hearing on the telephone?	YES___ NO___
Do I have a constant ringing or buzzing in my ears?	YES___ NO___
Do I often miss hearing the doorbell or a knock on the door?	YES___ NO___
Do I hear the turn signal in my car?	YES___ NO___
Does my family complain that I play the TV or radio too loud?	YES___ NO___
Do people complain that I don't pay attention to what they say?	YES___ NO___
Have I often been around loud noise?	YES___ NO___
Do members of my family have hearing problems?	YES___ NO___

Consider how your hearing has changed with the use of your hearing aids. Discuss your responses with your family and friends, if you wish, and compare the above results with those from your initial test. If your new hearing aids do not meet any of your expectations, discuss your concerns with your provider.

GOOD LUCK with YOUR hearing aid decision.

If you still have questions, here is a list of organizations that can provide you with additional information.

American Academy of Audiology
11730 Plaza America Drive
Suite 300
Reston, VA 20190
1-800- 222-2336
www.audiology.org

American Academy of Otolaryngology-Head and Neck Surgery, Inc
One Prince Street
Alexandria, VA 22314
703-836-4444
www.entnet.org

American Speech-Language-Hearing Association
10801 Rockville Pike
Rockville, MD 20852
1-800-638-8255
www.asha.org

American Tinnitus Association
P.O. Box 5
Portland, OR 97207
1-800-634-8978
www.ata.org

Better Hearing Institute
515 King Street
Suite 420
Alexandria, VA 22314
703-684-3391
www.betterhearing.org

Hearing Loss Association of America (formerly SHHH)
7910 Woodmont Avenue
Suite 1200
Bethesda, MD 20814
301-657-2248
www.hearingloss.org

International Hearing Society
16880 Middlebelt Road
Suite 4
Livonia, MI 48154
734-522-7200
www.ihsinfo.org

Citations

Kochkin, Sergei, MarkeTrak VII: Hearing Loss Population Tops 31 Million People, Hearing Review. 2005; Volume 12, No 7: pgs 16-29.

About the Authors

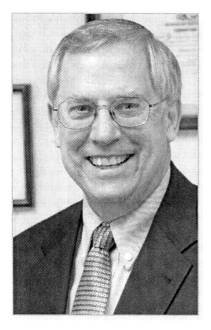

Randall D. Smith, M.Ed., has focused his career on helping individuals with communication problems. He has worked as a speech and hearing consultant, taught in a university setting, worked in a hospital speech and hearing clinic and currently owns his own practice. As a certified speech-language pathologist and a board certified hearing instrument specialist, Smith has worked with people with speech and hearing problems. He strives to understand each individual's personal communication issues and suggest options that best meet their needs. He wrote the predecessor to this book, *About Hearing Aids and Hearing Loss*, as well as numerous articles on practice management under managed care. He has lectured in university and professional settings on speech, language, and hearing problems. Smith's volunteer activities include work with the Developmental Disability Resource Center in Lakewood CO, InterFaith Community Services' Gift of Hearing Program, HearNow and SERTOMA.

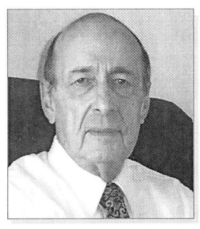

Jerome G. Alpiner, Ph.D., has devoted his professional career to helping children and adults hear better. He has done this through his involvement in university audiology programs, medical centers, and private practice. Dr. Alpiner has authored more than 100 articles, books, and book chapters dealing primarily with the rehabilitative audiological aspects of hearing. This includes hearing aids, auditory training, speechreading and counseling. He has spent considerable time working with the older population. Dr. Alpiner has also served as president and vice president of various organizations. He is a Fellow of the American Speech-Language-Hearing Association and was granted the Award of Honor of the Academy of Rehabilitative Audiology for his efforts in hearing. At present, he is a volunteer with Friends of Man, an organization that provides assistance to those in need.

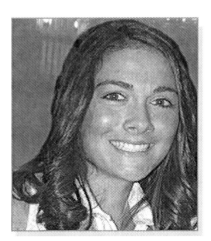

Megan Mulvey is currently pursuing her Doctor of Audiology degree at Rush University in Chicago. She has a Bachelor's Degree from the University of Iowa in Speech and Hearing Science. After obtaining her degree, she hopes to pursue a career in Pediatric Audiology and perform clinical research.

Notes:

Notes:

CORE COLLECTION 2008

Printed in the United States
202741BV00005B/43/A

9 780962 889103